D1724473

back stabilization and core strengthening

TABLE OF CONTENTS

The deep muscles of your stomach and low back are the core muscles of your body. They support and protect your low back and also help your leg and arm muscles work well. Doing the exercises in this booklet will strengthen your core muscles.

Please read the instructions and follow the advice of your doctor or physical therapist when you start or progress to more difficult exercises.

There are 4 basic starting positions:
- Hook-lying
- Face-down lying
- Hands and knees
- Bridge

The exercises get progressively more challenging in each position. Do not move to the next exercise in a series if you can't do the one before it. If your symptoms get worse while doing these exercises, talk to your doctor or physical therapist.

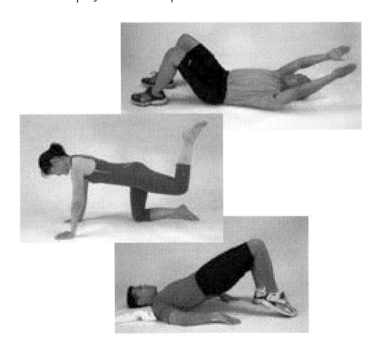

NEUTRAL POSITION

Lie on your back with your knees bent and your feet flat on the floor, which is the "hook-lying" position.

This is the starting position for the hook-lying exercises in this series. Find your **neutral position** by gently arching and flattening your back until you find a position where you are most comfortable. This is your **neutral position.** Gently tighten your stomach muscles without moving your back out of **neutral position**.

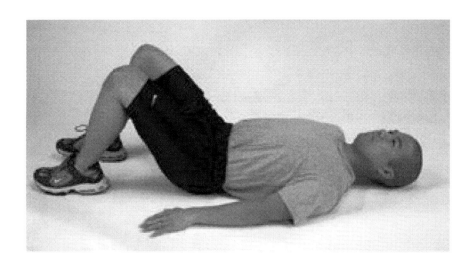

HOOK-LYING WITH ARM MOVEMENTS

Lie on your back with your knees bent and arms by your sides.

Find and hold your **neutral position** throughout the exercise.

A. One arm: Lift one arm overhead slowly. Return it to the start position while lifting the other arm overhead slowly. Continue by alternating right and left sides.

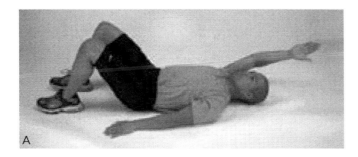

B. Both arms: Lift both arms overhead and return slowly to the start position while keeping your **neutral position.**

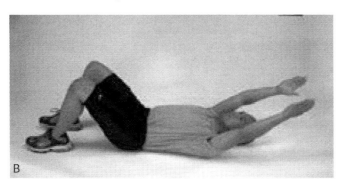

Do: A _____ B _____ Frequency _____

3

BENT KNEE TO SIDE

A. One knee bent: Lie on your back with one knee bent and the other leg straight. Find and hold your **_neutral position_** throughout the exercise. Slowly let your bent knee move out to the side without moving your other hip.

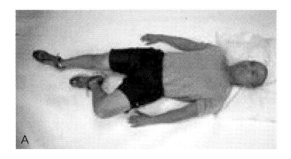

B. Both knees bent: Progress by doing the same exercise with both knees bent. Continue by alternating right and left sides.

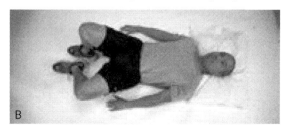

Do: A _____ B _____ Frequency _____

HEEL SLIDES

Lie on your back with your knees bent and your feet flat on the floor. Find and hold your **neutral position** throughout the exercise.

A. Heel slide: Keep your heel on the ground and slowly slide your foot forward until your leg is almost straight. Return to the start position by sliding your heel back. Repeat the movement with your other leg.

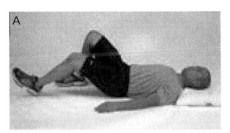

B. Heel lift and slide: Repeat exercise A with your heel lifted 1 to 2 inches from the floor. Continue by alternating right and left sides.

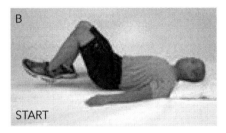

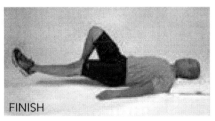

Do: A _____ B _____ Frequency _____

BENT KNEE LEG LIFT (SMALL STEPS)

Lie on your back with your knees bent and your feet flat on the floor. Find and hold your **neutral position** throughout the exercise.

A. One leg: Slowly lift one foot about 3 to 5 inches from the floor. Lower slowly. Repeat with the other foot and continue alternating legs as if taking small steps.

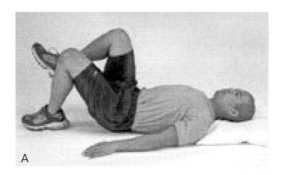

B. Both legs: Slowly lift one foot about 3 to 5 inches from the floor. Hold that position as you bring your other foot up. Slowly lower one leg, then the other. Continue this pattern: lift, lift, lower, lower.

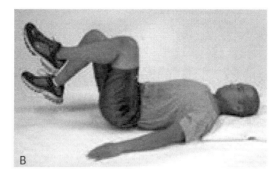

Do: A _____ B _____ Frequency _____

ALTERNATE ARM AND LEG LIFT

Lie on your back with your knees bent and your feet flat on the floor. Find and hold your **neutral position** throughout the exercise.

Slowly lift one arm overhead and lift your opposite foot 3 to 5 inches up from the floor. Slowly lower your arm and foot back to the floor. Repeat with your other arm and leg. Continue to alternate sides.

Frequency _____

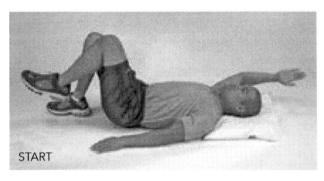

START

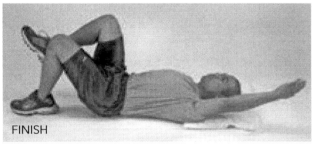

FINISH

CURL-UP

Lie on your back with your knees bent and your feet flat on the floor. Find and hold your **neutral position** throughout the exercise. Do not do this exercise if you have osteoporosis (thinning bones).

A. Hands on thigh: Place your hands on your thighs. Gently tighten your stomach muscles. Slowly lift your shoulders as you slide your hands toward your knees. Keep your neck muscles relaxed by holding your chin tucked in. Return to the start position.

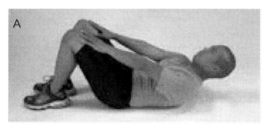

B. Hands behind head: Place your hands behind your head. Gently tighten your stomach muscles. Slowly lift your shoulders up from the floor. Support your neck with your hands but do not pull on your head. Return to the start position.

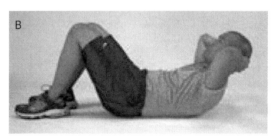

Do: A _____ B _____ Frequency _____

CURL-UP WITH ROTATION

Lie on your back with your knees bent and your feet flat on the floor. Find and hold your **neutral position** throughout the exercise. Do not do this exercise if you have osteoporosis (thinning bones).

A. One hand behind head: Place one hand behind your head. Gently tighten your stomach muscles. Lift your shoulder and reach with your free hand toward the opposite knee.

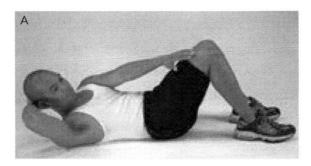

B. Both hands behind head: Place both hands behind your head. Gently tighten your stomach muscles. Lift one shoulder and bring it toward the opposite knee. Support your neck with your hands but do not pull on your head. Return to the start position.

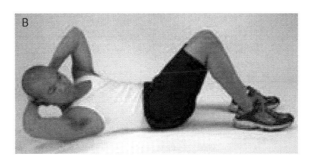

Do: A _____ B _____ Frequency _____

NEUTRAL POSITION

This is the starting position for the hands and knees exercises in this series. Get on your hands and knees. Your hands should be directly below your shoulders and your knees should be directly below your hips. Find your **neutral position** by gently moving your back up and down until you find the most comfortable position. Gently tighten your stomach muscles to hold your **neutral position.**

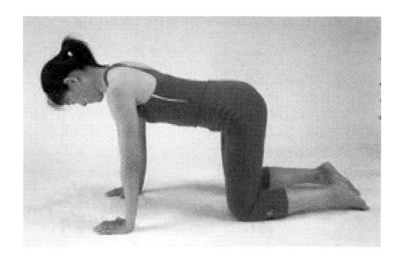

ROCKING FORWARD AND BACKWARD

Start on your hands and knees. Find and hold your **neutral position** throughout the exercise.

A. Rocking forward: Slowly move your body forward over your hands and then slowly return to the start position.

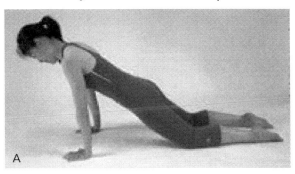

B. Rocking backward: Slowly move your body backward over your heels and then slowly return to the start position.

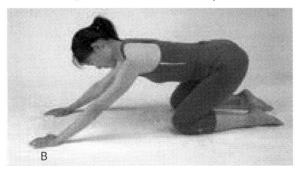

C. Rocking forward and backward: Combine exercise **A** and **B** by moving forward and backward in one smooth movement while maintaining your **neutral position.**

Do: A _____   B _____   C _____

Frequency _____

ARM SLIDE AND REACH

Start on your hands and knees. Find and hold your **neutral position** throughout the exercise.

A. Arm slide: Slowly slide one hand forward on the floor and then back to the start position. Repeat with your other side.

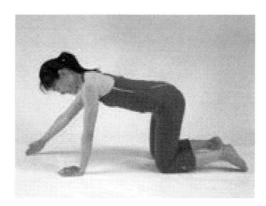

B. Arm reach: Lift one arm and reach forward. Slowly lower your arm to the start position. Repeat with the other arm, alternating sides.

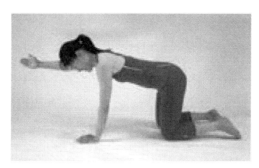

Do: A _____ B _____ Frequency _____

LEG SLIDE AND REACH

Start on your hands and knees. Find and hold your **neutral position** throughout the exercise.

A. Leg slide: Slide one leg back, keeping your toes on the floor. Return to the start position. Repeat with the other leg. Alternate sides.

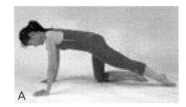

B. Leg lift—bent knee: Lift one leg 3 to 5 inches from the floor with your knee bent. Slowly lower leg to the start position. Repeat with the other leg. Continue alternating sides.

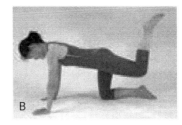

C. Leg reach: Slide one leg backward until the knee is straight. Lift your straight leg 3 to 5 inches from the floor. Slowly lower to the start position. Repeat with the other leg. Continue alternating

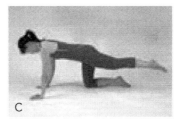

Do: A _____ B _____ C _____

Frequency _____

OPPOSITE ARM AND LEG SLIDE AND REACH

Start on your hands and knees. Find and hold your **neutral position** throughout the exercise.

A. Arm and leg slide: Slowly slide one leg backward keeping your toes on the floor. Slide your opposite arm forward at the same time. Return to the start position. Repeat with the other leg and arm. Continue alternating sides.

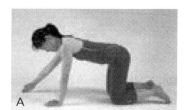

B. Arm slide with bent knee lift: Slowly lift one leg keeping your knee bent. Slide your opposite hand forward at the same time. Return to the start position. Repeat with the other leg and arm. Continue alternating sides.

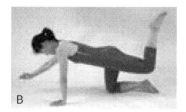

C. Arm and leg reach: Slowly slide one leg backward keeping your toes on the floor. Lift your foot 3 to 5 inches from the floor. At the same time, slide your opposite arm forward and lift 3 to 5 inches from the floor. Return to the start position. Repeat with the other leg and arm. Continue alternating sides.

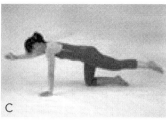

Do: A _____ B _____ C _____

Frequency _____

NEUTRAL POSITION

This is the starting position for the face-down stabilization exercises in this series. Lie on your stomach with your forehead resting on a small towel. Add a pillow under your stomach if it makes you more comfortable. Tighten your buttock muscles. This is your **neutral position**. You may feel a slight stretch in the front of your hips.

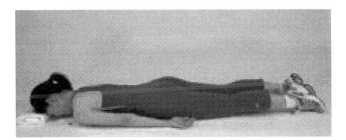

FACE-DOWN ONE-ARM LIFT

Start in the **neutral position** lying face down. Hold throughout the exercise. Stretch both arms above your head. With your thumb up, lift one arm 1-3 inches from the floor. Return to the start position and alternate arms.

Frequency _____

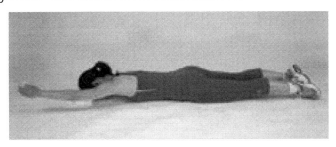

FACE-DOWN KNEE BEND/LIFT

Start in the **neutral position** lying face down. Hold throughout the exercise.

A. Knee bend: Bend one knee and then slowly lower your leg to the starting position. Repeat exercise with the other leg. Continue to alternate sides.

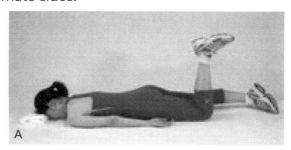

B. Knee bend and lift: Bend one knee. Tighten your buttocks muscles and lift your bent knee about 1 to 2 inches. Do not let your back move or arch. You may need a pillow under your hips to be able to do this exercise with good form. Hold for 5 seconds, and then lower your leg slowly to the start position. Repeat exercise with your other leg.

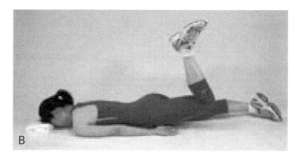

Do: A _____ B _____ Frequency _____

FACE-DOWN ARM/LEG LIFT

Start in the **neutral position** lying face down. Hold throughout the exercise.

A. **Leg lift:** Tighten your buttocks muscles and lift one straight leg 1 to 2 inches off the floor. Do not let your back arch. You may need to place a pillow under your hips to be able to do this exercise with good form. Hold for 5 seconds. Lower your leg slowly to the start position. Repeat exercise with your other leg.

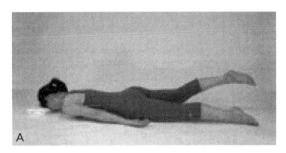

B. **Arm and leg lift:** Tighten your buttocks muscles. Lift one arm and your opposite leg 1 to 2 inches off the floor. Do not allow your back to twist or arch. Hold for 5 seconds and then lower your arm and leg to the start position. Repeat exercise with your other arm and leg.

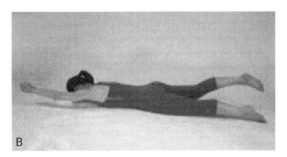

Do: A _____ B _____ Frequency _____

17

BASIC BRIDGE

This is the starting position for the bridge stabilization exercises in this series. Lie on your back with your knees bent and feet flat on the floor, hands by your sides. Gently tighten your stomach muscles. Lift your hips 3-5 inches from the floor without arching your back. Hold bridge for _____ seconds, and then slowly lower your hips to the floor.

Frequency _____

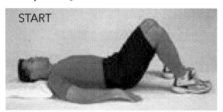
START

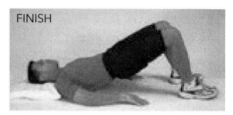
FINISH

BRIDGE WITH ARM LIFT

Start with a *Basic Bridge* and maintain this position throughout the exercise.

A. One arm lift: Hold the bridge position and move one arm overhead and back to your side. Alternate your arms, continuing to hold the bridge.

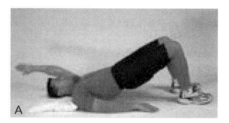
A

B. Both arms lift: Hold the bridge position and move both arms overhead and back to your sides.

Do: A _____   B _____

Frequency

_____

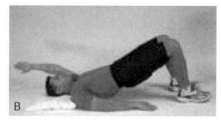
B

BRIDGE WITH LEG LIFT

Start with a **Basic Bridge** and maintain this position throughout the exercise.

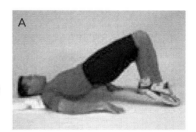

A. Heel lift: Lift one heel up keeping your toes on the floor. Slowly lower your heel to the floor. Repeat on the other side. Continue alternating while holding the bridge.

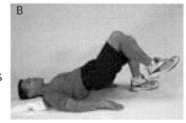

B. Marching: Lift one foot 3 to 5 inches, keeping your knee bent. Slowly lower your foot to the floor and repeat with the other side. Continue alternating as if marching in place.

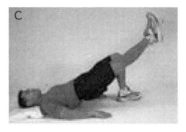

C. Leg lifts: lift one leg with your knee bent, and then straighten your knee. Hold ___ seconds. Slowly bend your knee and lower your leg, returning to the **Basic Bridge** position. Repeat the movement with the other leg. Continue alternating sides while holding the bridge.

Do: A _____   B _____   C _____

Frequency _____

19

SIDE SUPPORT PLANK

A. On knees: Lie on one side with both of your knees bent and your hips in line with your shoulders. Support your weight on

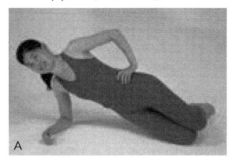

your forearm with your elbow directly under your shoulder. Rest your top hand on your hip. Tighten your stomach and buttocks muscles and keep them tight throughout the exercise. Lift your hips 3-4 inches from the floor. Hold _____ seconds. Slowly lower to the start position.

Frequency _____

Progress to holding _____ seconds

B. On Feet. Lie on your side with your knees, hips, and shoulders in line. Rest your top hand on your hip. Tighten your stomach

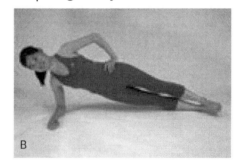

and buttocks muscles and keep them tight throughout the exercise. Lift your hips 3-4 inches from the floor. Keep your knees straight during this exercise. Hold _____ seconds. Slowly lower to the start position.

Frequency _____

Progress to holding _____ seconds

FACE-DOWN PLANK

A. On knees: Lie face down with your weight supported on your forearms and knees. Make sure your elbows are directly under your shoulders. You may cross your ankles. Tighten your stomach and buttocks muscles and keep them tight throughout the exercise.

Hold _____ seconds.

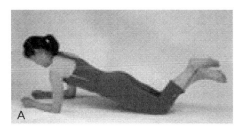

Frequency _____

Progress to holding _____ seconds

B. On feet: Lie face down with your weight supported on your toes and forearms. Tighten your stomach and buttocks muscles and keep them tight throughout the exercise. Do not let your back sag. Hold _____ seconds. Slowly lower your knees to the ground.

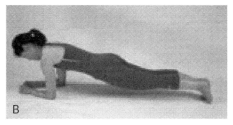

Frequency _____

Progress to holding _____ seconds

Exercise Diary

It sometimes helps to keep an **exercise diary**. This will remind you when you last did your exercises and is a place to note anything you want to remember or if you are part of an exercise group, you may want to share with your Chair based Exercise Leader.

Date (eg. Monday 2nd January)	Comments (eg. Did not do a specific exercise, feel you have improved doing a particular exercise)

Exercise Diary

It sometimes helps to keep an **exercise diary**. This will remind you when you last did your exercises and is a place to note anything you want to remember or if you are part of an exercise group, you may want to share with your Chair based Exercise Leader.

Date (eg. Monday 2nd January)	Comments (eg. Did not do a specific exercise, feel you have improved doing a particular exercise)

Exercise Diary

It sometimes helps to keep an **exercise diary**. This will remind you when you last did your exercises and is a place to note anything you want to remember or if you are part of an exercise group, you may want to share with your Chair based Exercise Leader.

Date (eg. Monday 2nd January)	Comments (eg. Did not do a specific exercise, feel you have improved doing a particular exercise)

Exercise Diary

It sometimes helps to keep an **exercise diary**. This will remind you when you last did your exercises and is a place to note anything you want to remember or if you are part of an exercise group, you may want to share with your Chair based Exercise Leader.

Date (eg. Monday 2nd January)	Comments (eg. Did not do a specific exercise, feel you have improved doing a particular exercise)

Exercise Diary

It sometimes helps to keep an **exercise diary**. This will remind you when you last did your exercises and is a place to note anything you want to remember or if you are part of an exercise group, you may want to share with your Chair based Exercise Leader.

Date (eg. Monday 2nd January)	Comments (eg. Did not do a specific exercise, feel you have improved doing a particular exercise)

Exercise Diary

It sometimes helps to keep an **exercise diary**. This will remind you when you last did your exercises and is a place to note anything you want to remember or if you are part of an exercise group, you may want to share with your Chair based Exercise Leader.

Date (eg. Monday 2nd January)	Comments (eg. Did not do a specific exercise, feel you have improved doing a particular exercise)

Exercise Diary

It sometimes helps to keep an **exercise diary**. This will remind you when you last did your exercises and is a place to note anything you want to remember or if you are part of an exercise group, you may want to share with your Chair based Exercise Leader.

Date (eg. Monday 2nd January)	Comments (eg. Did not do a specific exercise, feel you have improved doing a particular exercise)

Exercise Diary

It sometimes helps to keep an **exercise diary**. This will remind you when you last did your exercises and is a place to note anything you want to remember or if you are part of an exercise group, you may want to share with your Chair based Exercise Leader.

Date (eg. Monday 2nd January)	Comments (eg. Did not do a specific exercise, feel you have improved doing a particular exercise)

Exercise Diary

It sometimes helps to keep an **exercise diary**. This will remind you when you last did your exercises and is a place to note anything you want to remember or if you are part of an exercise group, you may want to share with your Chair based Exercise Leader.

Date (eg. Monday 2nd January)	Comments (eg. Did not do a specific exercise, feel you have improved doing a particular exercise)

Exercise Diary

It sometimes helps to keep an **exercise diary**. This will remind you when you last did your exercises and is a place to note anything you want to remember or if you are part of an exercise group, you may want to share with your Chair based Exercise Leader.

Date (eg. Monday 2nd January)	Comments (eg. Did not do a specific exercise, feel you have improved doing a particular exercise)

Exercise Diary

It sometimes helps to keep an **exercise diary**. This will remind you when you last did your exercises and is a place to note anything you want to remember or if you are part of an exercise group, you may want to share with your Chair based Exercise Leader.

Date (eg. Monday 2nd January)	Comments (eg. Did not do a specific exercise, feel you have improved doing a particular exercise)

Exercise Diary

It sometimes helps to keep an **exercise diary**. This will remind you when you last did your exercises and is a place to note anything you want to remember or if you are part of an exercise group, you may want to share with your Chair based Exercise Leader.

Date (eg. Monday 2nd January)	Comments (eg. Did not do a specific exercise, feel you have improved doing a particular exercise)

Printed in France by Amazon
Brétigny-sur-Orge, FR

20080458R00022